THE HARD GAINER
REPORT

By Greg Sushinsky

www.gregsushinsky.com

Contents

Who is a Hard Gainer?

You are, if you are thin, skinny, underweight, have a difficult time putting on muscle or even gaining a small amount of bodyweight, or are not particularly strong--then you are most likely a hard gainer. While so many people around you are busy--or even obsessed--with trying to lose weight, you are continually trying to gain, or secretly wish you had the problem of weight to lose, or perhaps you have even given up trying to gain weight and muscle size. Maybe you feel you have tried every type of workout, every type of diet; you've tried to lift enormous poundages (for you) which are beyond your strength, yet still your bodybuilding results are, by your own standards, close to zero. Don't give up, don't despair. If you have given up, try again, but this time we will show you ways you can utilize to reach your goals, so finally you'll have a chance to achieve your dreams of greater muscle size and strength.

HOPE

There is hope for you as a hard gainer. You need not resign yourself to an unhappy outcome that you won't ever have a chance at improving your size and strength. You can, if you apply yourself with hard work, care and intelligence, probably realize substantial gains in muscle size and strength. While it's true that nobody can know the eventual outcome of your size and strength potential, as this is a matter genetically conditioned, it can be seen as a challenge instead of a condemnation to have lower initial potential or more obstacles in your bodybuilding. Others in the past have succeeded, some mightily, in overcoming a seeming tremendous lack of potential, and have become hard gainers who have made good, and some, even great gains. While nobody can rightly guarantee you results, if you learn to apply what we teach you in this report, you may make surprising gains.

Preliminaries: HEALTH

Before we get underway with a discussion of the key hard gainer elements such as nutrition and training, we should mention something about health. Prior to considering how you will go about your bodybuilding, you need to ascertain your general health. Are you in good general health? Perhaps you can best assess this by asking yourself a few simple questions: Do you have ample energy, or are you easily fatigued or tired much of the time? The greater your energy, the more and harder you'll be able to work out. Are you physically active or not?

If you're more active, used to working out, you'll be able to adapt to the workouts more readily than if you've been relatively inactive. Do you have allergies or any medical conditions? Allergies, including food allergies, may necessitate that you make certain modifications in your diet; medications may alter how you feel during or after workouts, or may affect your appetite. Have you had surgeries which might prevent you from doing certain exercises? If so, there are ways of learning to work around this by choosing other exercises. Is your work or normal daily activity physical and strenuous, or sedentary?

This, along with the earlier question about overall physical activity, is a factor in what you can do in your workouts. A sedentary job will allow you to recover more from workouts, whereas a physical one (say, construction work) will make it more difficult to do so. What are your eating habits? Do you eat nutritious foods, or lots of junk foods? This will be a significant factor in your rate of progress. The better your nutrition, the better your chance of progress. Are you a disciplined or erratic eater? Same thing here. Disciplined eaters do better; the body comes to expect a certain pattern in eating and digestion. And there might be many more ways of looking at your health profile, but this gives you an idea of how to think about it.

All these kinds of questions can assist you in determining how you are going to approach your hard gainer bodybuilding. This self-inventory can help you figure out how to best apply the information and suggestions for your hard gainer training and nutrition. Your own answers on the self-inventory questions can help identify what potential problem areas you might have, how you can hope to solve them, and what personal boundaries or limitations you may need to take note of and work within.

Your answers may also point up potentially strong points of which you weren't previously aware. Whatever your thoughts on the self-inventory, there's certainly no need to memorize it, nor is there even a need to dwell on your answers, but it is a tool you can use or return to so as to help you in your quest for better results.

More preliminaries: MEDICAL

If you must maintain a special diet, for example, for medical reasons, you need to keep this in mind when you are studying the section on nutrition and trying to implement the suggestions. If you have trouble digesting certain foods (dairy products, for example), you'll have to factor that into your dietary approach. If you have a chronic disease or disability, (digestive or otherwise) you should also work with your physician or other health professional to take this into consideration when undergoing a program of bodybuilding and nutrition as a hard gainer. One further note about medical conditions or disabilities: many people have worked around and through such situations to achieve their greatest potential still, in spite of the limitations, so this should encourage you.

METABOLISM

For bodybuilding purposes, consider a basic understanding of metabolism as the sum total of physiological processes that relate to processing food and creating energy in the body, for our purposes here ultimately culminating in building muscle and diminishing fat. One of the keys to successful bodybuilding, especially in the case of hard gainers, is to be able to match your training and nutrition to your metabolic needs. Hard gainers, as we have said, often have the kind of metabolism that burns up calories at a rapid rate, so gaining weight and muscle is often a great struggle. So one of the concepts necessary for hard gainers to understand is the attempt to bring the metabolic rate down slightly, to help gain weight and muscle size.

While people tend to have a metabolic rate which seems set in a genetic range over their lifetime, some alteration, at least temporary, is desirable for hard gainers and is possible through the application of exercise, nutrition and rest. This is a critical area for any hard gainer. So keep in mind that much of the hard gainer nutrition and training information in this report is designed with the understanding that implementing the information will automatically go along with also getting the metabolism to operate at an optimum rate for hard gainer muscle growth.

I. NUTRITION

1. EATING

This is almost certainly what you need to do more of. You simply need to find a way to ingest more good calories--nutritious food--to go with your training. Though this seems utterly simplistic, many hard gainers don't realize this, let alone know how to do it. Sometimes, there are debates in bodybuilding about the role and importance of nutrition, whether it makes up a certain percentage of importance, whether it is primary or secondary to training in importance, whether it is all important or not important at all, but in the case of hard gainers, eating well, and often more than you currently do, is even more important than your training, as important as your training is.

Why is this so? Training stimulates or promotes muscle growth in a complex, indirect way, but ultimately only in the presence of other factors, one of which is at least adequate--and usually more than adequate--nutrients. Let's suppose you are a 5'8" male, weighing 125 pounds. For bodybuilding purposes, if you wish to gain 20 or 30 pounds of mostly muscle, even if you work out like a demon, but are taking in fewer calories than you are expending, you will end up losing weight and perhaps even muscle mass, rather than gaining. This scenario, unfortunately, does occur with many hard gainers, who may not know where to turn, so they eventually abandon their efforts.   If you're in such a situation, don't.

Some hard gainers understand the importance of eating consistently and eating sufficient calories, but they don't know how to put this into practice. They often overestimate the amount of calories they are eating at the time, or fail to understand that they sometimes must dramatically increase this to get the body to respond. An example of this is if someone weighs 150 pounds, and they have determined by a common general formula (such as a rough rule that you need to take in about 10 or 12 calories per pound of bodyweight to maintain your present bodyweight) that they need in the neighborhood of 2,000 calories a day just to maintain that bodyweight, and they feel if they add minimal calories, going up to 2,050 or even 2,100, they should gain. Yet often they fail to gain weight on this calorie increase. Why?

The mathematical formulas you often read about regarding adequate calorie intake are generalizations. You may hear you only need 12 calories per pound of bodyweight to maintain your weight, or 10 calories, or some such figure. But in our example, the 150 pound hard gainer clearly needs at least 13 calories per pound (i.e., 2,000 calories divided by 150 pounds bodyweight), and might need at least 15 calories per pound of bodyweight just to maintain that 150 pounds. And, at least for some time, he will have to eat more than this amount to gain. Actually the emphasis shouldn't be on the math, but on the eating. Yet common formulas will advise such a hard gainer if he increases his calories by only a few per day (as little as 10 or 15), he'll gain weight and it will be all muscle, not fat. This is theory--unhelpful theory at that. It can keep hard gainers from achieving their goals and can cause them to give up.

2. How to Gain Weight

In the case of our 150 pound hard gainer, and most real-world trainees, he might have to try to eat significantly more calories than the slight amounts suggested over and above the theoretical maintenance levels. This could be something in the range of a total of 2,500 to 3,000 calories per day as opposed to the 2,000 he was eating previously, and in some cases, perhaps even as much as 4,000 (or 5,000) calories or more a day for a short period of time, to gain substantially. Why? Because the body is going to resist change, for one thing, and for another, people who respond well to smaller increments or decrements in daily calorie changes, simply have more responsive metabolisms than most hard gainers. Now this increase is not necessary initially or all at once, but it illustrates where the hard gainer may have to aim his eventual nutritional intake goals.

An important point to remember: The hard gainer in our example should not, in any event, attempt to jump from his 2,000 calories to 2,500, 3,000 or 4,000-5,000 all at once. The higher amount of calories simply illustrates the task and how, eventually, it might be worked out. Adding 50 or 100 calories at a time—gradually--is always best. The point is that the hard gainer probably needs to keep at it, to keep these small calorie increases progressive and cumulative. Weeks, months and a couple of years would be the safest, healthiest, and most effective means of doing this.

The 4,000 or more calorie figure might only be necessitated as the hard gainer becomes larger and gains weight along months or a couple of years. Or, eating regularly and boosting the calories over the baseline figure which is as low as the 2,000 by a lesser (say, several hundred additional calories) but consistent amount over months could do it. But simply eating a couple hundred calories a day extra for only a week or two likely will not. Consistently applying a gradual approach, giving your body time to adjust--this is always better in your nutritional approach.

Let's do some more math. Keep looking at the theories out there today which have misled hard gainers. By formula, adding an extra 1,000 calories per day--admittedly a large and sometimes difficult increase for many hard gainers--would add 7,000 calories per week, which supposedly equates, according to critics, to two pounds of added bodyfat per week. (The operative theoretical math being that it takes approximately 3,500 calories to equal a pound of fat as against approximately 500-700 calories to equal a pound of muscle gain.) But what happens if a hard gainer is able to achieve the often difficult task of adding significant calories to his or her diet? They almost never gain fat, they often gain muscle instead, sometimes a little, sometimes a lot. This process, again, in the human body, does not always work in such a predictable way, but it is an attempt to illustrate that hard gainers, who seldom begin getting fat on any kind of calorie increase, need to have a different approach to their eating and nutrition than do others.

So how do you go about gaining the muscle size and the bodyweight you want? Eating, as we indicated, is a huge key. For some hard gainers--extreme or severe hard gainers, the question might be, how do you even gain a pound? And this is no exaggeration--some hard gainers have not and feel they are unable to gain weight at all, and feel they cannot ever, but in most cases they can. Or at least they will be able to eventually. Adjusting the food intake is the key, and once they gain the first additional pound of bodyweight and muscle mass, they can keep applying the principles that give them the greatest chance of success.

More Food

Many nutritionists are horrified by the practice of a large increase in calories that some hard gainers undertake. Many hard gainers, on the other hand, are eager and intrigued as to how to do it. They understand or come to understand, through lack of previous success, of their need to increase their calorie intake, and they may say, "bring on the food," but then before even getting to the eating part, are puzzled as to what to eat.

What do you eat if you want to gain weight, a small or great amount of muscle? Are there special foods? Secret foods? The best news is that ordinary available foods can and have been the staple of drug-free hard gainers over the course of decades of the history of bodybuilding. You can concentrate on good sources of protein such as eggs, milk, beef, chicken, turkey, fish, along with carbohydrates such as a wide range of vegetables, fruits, breads, whole grains, and of course the staple carbohydrates (starches) such as potatoes, pasta and rice. This list is obviously not exhaustive. Include some fats now regarded as health-promoting such as olive oil, fish oil or flax seed oil, or take in essential fatty acids (EFAs).

Yes, you should include some amount of animal fats as they occur in your diet. The types of foods that made up the majority of successful hard gainer nutrition years ago were beef, eggs, and milk, along with other meats, vegetables, starches and fruits, eaten in ample quantities. Many of these foods--beef, eggs and milk--of course, contain animal fats. Yes, it sounds heretical, given today's nutritional edicts against just those foods.

In sufficient quantities, though, coupled with proper training, the inclusion of beef, eggs, and milk, which formed the core of hard gainer nutrition, resulted in bodyweight, muscle and strength gains, often along with improved health, but that part is a more subjective outcome.

There is a problem, though. Many bodybuilding nutritionists, for reasons that are too complicated to go into detail here, now recommend the low fat (or ultra low fat), high carbohydrate, moderate to low protein diet for all natural bodybuilders, including hard gainers. This has been disastrous for hard gainers. Setting aside the question of whether the current bodybuilding nutritional recommendations are the right ones for all natural bodybuilders, these recommendations are almost always wrong for hard gainers. The lack of beef, eggs, and milk--which from the 1930s or so up until the 1970s or

1980s actually, as we said,   functioned as the core of successful hard gainer nutrition, has taken the heart out of a nutritional approach that can be extremely beneficial for hard gainers. The campaign against such foods as beef, eggs, and milk, as being too fat laden and therefore unhealthy, has left hard gainers with a lesser arsenal to fight their cause.

Though it is certainly not proof, keep in mind that the hard gainers of decades past swore by the properties of beef, eggs, and milk--these now nearly condemned, sometimes forbidden foods--for both their health and their bodybuilding gains, often when nothing else worked. Anecdotal, true. Politically incorrect, very true. But worth considering all the same. Including these foods in the hard gainer's diet rather than completely excluding them, as many try to do, usually leads to better muscle building results.

MUSCLE FOODS

Strictly speaking, there are no such foods that when eaten, guarantee that they will "turn into" muscle on the human body. That said, there are some ways of eating which do seem to promote the greater chance of gaining muscular bodyweight than others. In the ancient hard gainer days before anabolic steroids, as we already indicated, foods such as beef, eggs, and milk were invested with almost mystical powers for promoting muscle and strength.

Because we are more "enlightened" now, and we eat mostly (or only) lowfat fare such as chicken, fish, turkey or meals consisting largely if not completely of carbohydrates, we should be seeing better results and better health. But in the case of hard gainers, as far as bodyweight, muscle and strength gains, we are not. One reason is simply calories: a pound of various cuts of beef can contain around 1,000 calories, whereas a pound of tuna fish, for example, may have approximately 500 calories. While the fish has nutritive value, first things first: it's harder to get the calories on the lowfat diet.

This is not to recommend exclusive beef eating versus fish or chicken--by all means you should include those great foods--but it does show that on a calorie and food volume basis alone, beef has something positive to offer the hard gainer. He might instead include the beef, and alternate or rotate eating the various meat proteins, such as beef, fish, chicken, or turkey.

Of course the big objection most nutritionists have to beef is twofold: 1). Too many calories in beef (which is just what the hard gainers need and want!) 2) And the value of the nutrients from the fish or beef is disputed. Fish--and let's say again fish can be a very good, healthful, beneficial food, even included for hard gainers--does not have what beef has. Its critics will say yes, it does not have the fat (though some kinds of fish do have fat), that beef has. Often true, yet the fat is a way of delivering calories and needed fats to the usually calorie and fat-starved hard gainer.

The fats in beef can contribute to the all-important promotion of hormone production, so essential in muscle and strength growth. Hormone production and muscle growth in the hard gainer would be likely to long occur before any of the potentially damaging effects of excessive animal fats would occur in the diet of the hard gainer. When he has such a vast deficiency of calories and eating large amounts of food is notably difficult, beef can deliver a great deal of badly needed calories and nutrients to the hard gainer.

3. MAXIMIZED EATING (Calorie & Volume Dense Food)

The nutritional strategy you need to employ as a hard gainer could be summed up in the phrase "maximized eating," which is simply a way of saying that you need to get the most bodybuilding efficiency for your calories, food volume, and the kinds of food you eat. Thus, you can design your own eating plans which take into account your particular preferences as well as the uniqueness of your body. If, for example, you are able to eat lots of good, health-promoting food without feeling stuffed or bloated, and you are gaining weight, muscle size and strength, and you are doing this with lots of "white meat" (i.e., chicken, fish, turkey, as opposed to beef or "red meat"), and you enjoy this nutritional approach, then continue doing it. But for most of you, at least including some beef, milk and eggs, if you have no trouble digesting them, in an overall balanced nutritional program (meaning, don't neglect other nutritious foods such as vegetables, fruits, and starches in ample quantities) will, as we have pointed out, contribute to the calorie and nutrient efficiency we are striving for in setting up a maximized eating plan.

Also, liquid calories, such as those in fruit juices and milk, are an easy way for hard gainers to get calories down--simply drink them. While milk and fruit juices might be off limits to some dieters, these deliver easy calories, needed calories, for the body-starved hard gainer. Yes, everybody's different, including hard gainers--from each other. Ultimately, the individuality of your own body and its responses to nutrition and exercise should help you necessarily modify whatever nutrition and exercise you undertake. But keep the principle of maximized eating in mind.

DIGESTION

The heart of the nutritional matter for the hard gainer is not really eating so much as digestion and assimilation. We only eat as a means to an end in terms of ultimately providing our bodies with what they need in the way of nutrients, calories, and so on. So to enhance digestion, you can attempt to utilize the practice of eating several smaller meals, usually as many as six (though there's no magic in this number) instead of three. Now this doesn't have to mean necessarily that these six meals--or feedings--are all traditional in terms of size and scope. They actually could consist of the more traditional three meals of breakfast, lunch and dinner with three snacks interspersed.

These additional snacks/meals could consist of whatever you are eating on your hard gainer plan, but what is usually included is at least some small amount of protein, along with something additional. Some cheese and an apple, for instance, could make up one such snack. Or a sandwich. Tuna, or hot or cold chicken or roast beef, or any meat of your choice might make a good sandwich. Add a side of vegetables or potatoes, pasta or rice. Use your microwave. Save and eat your leftovers, they're valuable to you. Learn to cook some simple, basic stuff which you can refrigerate or freeze and eat later. Do whatever's convenient and effective.

The particulars are easy to figure out once you understand the plan, which is to spread your daily eating out over a greater number of meals for digestive comfort. You don't want to be forcing down more food than your system can handle, as this is counter productive to your goals. If before you even undertake any hard gainer nutrition plan you have digestive problems which restrict what you can eat, or for which you are under medical care, then of course you must follow those guidelines and adjust the kinds and amounts of food you can eat. This is not to say your program will be unsuccessful, though your results may not be as dramatic or as good as someone who can handle a wider range and amount of food. You'll have to be more patient, diligent, and careful, that's all.

If six meals are impractical for you--and they often are, as most people work, go to school, or have other demands on their schedules--then don't worry about this and simply adjust to as much food as you need via as many meals as you can comfortably eat within your hard gainer program. You may, again, have to reduce your expectations, though it is possible you may not. The six meal plan, which has its roots in some of the original, old-time, successful hard gainer nutrition plans, has become a part of modern bodybuilding orthodoxy, so much so that people feel if they can't do six meals a day, they can't really bodybuild. It's not true. Hard gainers also used to gain well on three meals or four, or even two meals a day.

You may have to compromise and come close to eating more than you might want in those meals, but for hard gainers who've been eating irregular meals and too lightly in the first place, even three normal-sized meals a day coupled with a good workout can ignite tremendous gains. Again, if you are restricted to or prefer three meals a day and you can eat enough and digest it comfortably, then stick with it. So do what you can realistically do, don't worry about what you can't do, and you'll be on your way to achieving your goals.

4. PROTEIN

One of the sometimes still controversial subjects in bodybuilding has to do with protein. The modern or post-modern bodybuilding nutritional theories often come down on the side of moderate or even low percentages of protein in the diet (as low as 15 or 20 percent), as such proponents insist that little, if any, additional protein is necessary to build muscle and to meet the body's demands for vigorous workouts. We wonder, however, as the pre-steroid nutrition era in bodybuilding suggested lots of protein--sometimes seemingly enormous amounts, (such as eating a gram or two or more per pound of bodyweight, on the order of 40% to 60% of total calories.) The history of success of hard gainers, though, is that additional amounts (though not necessarily gigantic amounts) over what the most conservative nutritionists recommend has often bought good results.

Even if, as in the case of calories and especially fats (but also carbohydrates), this style of eating is relatively temporary, say over a period of weeks or months until bodyweight and muscle size goals are achieved, and the hard gainer then resumes a more customary style of eating, with a more traditional balance between protein, carbohydrates and fats, the benefits of temporary protein increases are worth noting and trying, adjusted individually and of course in line with whatever personal health concerns exist. Protein increases work best for hard gainers, though, when they haven't been eating enough protein in the first place. Keep this also in mind.

Try it this way, if you wish to experiment: begin by gradually adding protein, whether with additional protein foods or protein powders (see upcoming supplements section), and note your response. You may want to add more protein if you feel it is helping bring about an increase in bodyweight, strength and muscle size, but you should always monitor how this feels. Some people simply don't want to eat a lot of protein; others can't; some people shouldn't. Health should rule over desire and even results. And there is this further information: most hard gainers need a basic increase in bodyweight (their most important task), and too much extra protein is not necessarily the most efficient way to do that. Often, sheer calories, with adequate protein, plenty of carbohydrates and sufficient fats are the route to go.

Simply adding lots of protein (or overdosing on it), especially when reducing the carbs and fats--especially a severe reduction of carbs and fats, may even cause weight loss, not weight gain. (Hard gainers should not reduce carbohydrate intake when trying to gain weight.) Protein is used more effectively as a central tool in weight reducing or fat loss dieting in this way, which is the opposite goal of hard gainers, as protein's properties are much more suited to weight loss or maintenance than weight gaining.

Carbohydrates and fats, calorie for calorie, via the way they are processed in the body, will contribute more toward gaining weight than protein will. (And must be included along with any protein increase to gain weight, as we said). So if you are eating a good balance of protein, carbohydrates and fats, simply adding more calories in every category will meet the task more effectively.

5. BULKING UP, EXTREME DIETS

The "protein flooding" style of nutrition for the hard gainer, which was touched upon in the last section, leads us to its close cousin, which is a much wider topic, that of bulking up. The ideal method of bulking up or gaining weight, especially for the hard gainer is, despite the terminology, more gradual than force feeding, more eating and digesting in relative comfort than jamming calories and food down until the very thought of eating again fills you with a feeling of revulsion. While we know historically some extreme force-feeding methods have been popular, and most of us have tried something like it (at least once, or perhaps once only being enough)--and while it's true that any kind of increased calorie eating may technically be considered a bulking up plan--usually the most lasting results are achieved by hard gainers undertaking the more gradual, consistent, long term approach we are outlining here.

Move your calories up in stages or increments, not all at once if you are attempting a great increase. Get your body (and especially your digestive processes) used to taking in more food. If you do happen to attempt a super increase in calories, a force feeding or near force-feeding plan (which, admittedly, while extreme and not recommended, has sometimes worked), at least put a time limit on it (preferably shorter rather than longer), or take breaks from this kind of eating periodically and at some point revert to a more normal, reasonable calorie level.

The same goes for you if you are going to undertake a relatively unbalanced program with a (temporary) emphasis on meat, milk, and eggs or other heavy ingestion of protein as some of the old timers did. If you want to try this, at least don't go overboard on it and keep a close eye on how you feel. You want to ensure your health and you want to make lasting bodybuilding gains, so make healthy bulking up--healthy weight gaining--not forced over-feeding, a part of your hard gainer plan. And again, don't just center on meats or proteins, include plenty of starches, fruits and vegetables. You want to stay healthy and gain, two compatible goals.

To reiterate, gradual, long term weight-gaining is the way to go; get your body used to slight increases in calories and food, and this will add up to the cumulative larger increases you may want over time. This is a solid, proven way to make good and even great gains. Try it and stick with it. And as mentioned, always continue to include other nutritious foods besides proteins; starches, plenty of vegetables and fruits, along with your meats are just as important to your health, well-being, and ultimately, your gains.

WATER

While technically not a nutrient or a food, you can't live without it. And you can't train well without it or have good health and muscle growth without it. Water is essential to human life, necessary in the human body, and necessary directly or indirectly to just about every physiological process that goes on inside of us. You should drink sufficient water. The old days (not that long ago, actually) where water was denied athletes, or athletes (including bodybuilders) would not drink water before, during or after training, either resulted in poor, inadequate (if not dangerously so) hydration, at the very least, or might have even compromised health and held back bodybuilding gains.

There is still no real consensus on hydrating, though more seems to be better. You needn't bloat yourself, but waiting until you are thirsty, particularly if you are physically active (and you are if you are weight training), is an invitation to be improperly hydrated, even dehydrated. So drink water before you are thirsty. Drink water throughout the day. You can drink other liquids, but simple unadulterated water is still the best way to hydrate. Don't neglect this seemingly obvious requirement.

SUPPLEMENTS

A word about supplements. Hard gainers, for a number of reasons, should first concentrate on improving their nutrition. That is, eating better food, eating more often, and eating enough for their goals. If a hard gainer has been eating two small meals per day consisting of nachos, fries, soda and pizza, then he has a long way to go to fix his nutrition for bodybuilding purposes. Where he is nutritionally at the moment, supplements would be pointless.

For the hard gainer who has eaten fairly well and has increased his calories properly, it still is better to concentrate on whole, real foods rather than supplements. The nutrients (and calories, don't forget--critical for hard gainers) available in real food are abundant and superior in most cases to what supplements have to offer. And while an in-depth discussion of food supplements is beyond the scope of our space here, a lot supplements have been historically over-hyped, overpriced, often ineffective, sometimes worthless, sometimes of minimal value, and sometimes have merely supplied ineffectively what you could get from real food.

That said, some additions, such as multi-vitamin minerals and related products, are often helpful. And protein supplements, which have the longest continuous successful use in bodybuilding history of any supplement, can be valuable. As we said previously, just don't go overboard on protein.   You can usually find relatively economical milk-and -egg and/or whey protein powders (and even soy, though it's wrongly been discarded by most bodybuilders) that can conveniently find a place into your nutrition schedule.

Desiccated liver is de-bunked by most modern bodybuilding experts, but it has a long, consistent history of positive results. Weight gain powders are not usually as beneficial, as they are often sugar-filled with inferior ingredients. Creatine has a more mixed success story, with its sometimes difficult to digest or assimilate characteristics (as well as its overuse). Meal replacements and nutrition bars are often less nutritive than the meals they are designed to replace, but as a compromise, may fit.

Necessity and convenience are legitimate factors to consider in your eating. Just remember that supplements are additions to your nutrition, so continue to improve your nutrition by centering on real food and slowly add supplements as you investigate, experiment and feel the need. But be wary of whatever the new wonder supplement of the day is; many of these are untested, unproven. Real food works. So center your nutritional approach on whole, relatively unprocessed, real food. To sum up your eating: remember, don't count calories. Eat them!

JUNK FOOD

We'll keep this short. In a perfect universe, none of us would eat things that were bad for us. Either that, or all foods that were available would be both great tasting and good for us. Our universe is not that way at all, so there are a lot of foods that either do bad things to us (and our bodybuilding) or don't add anything positive. Yet most of us, from time to time, indulge in forbidden foods, foods without nutritive value--candies, desserts, sodas, ice cream, you name it, we humans eat it. Bodybuilders too. Hard gainers also. Some of this won't hurt you; a lot of it will slow or undo your bodybuilding progress.

If you're living on pies, cakes, or whatever other devitalized (though strangely, often tasty) stuff you can imagine, then you've got a problem. For hard gainers, every calorie taken in should contribute something positive to your bodybuilding quest. Ideally strive to minimize the damage or lack of good you're doing when you eat some of this stuff, but the most important part of your nutrition is to focus on good nutritious food, so that the junk food habit will be diminished and not a meaningful factor in your nutrition.

Other Nutritional Approaches

The nutritional approach we have suggested begins with a kind of modified mainstream nutrition program. It utilizes common foods in our culture which are plentiful, readily available (at any grocery store), and fits in with the way most of us eat, or at least aspire to eat. There are, however, other ways. Though we recognize it is difficult and not the generally accepted path, there are hard gainers who for a number of personal reasons, religious reasons, ethical considerations, health, medical or cultural reasons, prefer and practice very different ways of nutrition. Vegetarian eating is one such way.

Though there are and have been successful vegetarian bodybuilders, there are many more who have tried and failed to be satisfied with their results, so if you are following such an approach, be apprised of its difficulty, far more so for the vegetarian hard gainer. Most of your nutrition will have to be structured to be able to still deliver the necessary muscle, strength and energy building nutrients via foods that are acceptable to you. The best thing to do is to consult someone in the vegetarian community who practices bodybuilding, preferably someone who also is conversant with hard gainer problems. This recommendation would go for any of the many other alternative nutritional approaches.

II. TRAINING

1. PHYSICAL BASE (Foundation)

We know you want to get right to the training, but it's important to have something to start with. You will probably be able to begin better and progress faster, at least initially, if you have some experience with physical activity in the way of a sport or exercise or any kind of fitness activity. Your general fitness level, in addition to your general health, is an underlying factor in your bodybuilding success, and especially for hard gainer bodybuilding. Though this is a mostly-neglected facet of training nowadays by both bodybuilders and trainers, it is extremely important. If you are completely sedentary, don't just jump into a vigorous weight-training or bodybuilding program, even a program tailored to the hard gainer. Ease into it. Weight training is a much more intensive activity than even many sports, exercise or fitness activities, so take this into account.

If you can curb your eagerness to begin, perhaps take a couple of weeks (at least) to work on basic calisthenics, or exercises of your choice. Something that gets your body slightly used to the rigors of working out--any kind of working out--will be good. You can do this two or three times a week, or even daily for a while if you don't overdo it. Perhaps you can run instead of or in addition to some calisthenics, or swim or hike or ride a bike or play a sport--or anything else you can think of to do along these lines--practically any physical activity that you can do vigorously will be beneficial, and will prepare you for the challenge of weight-training.

Even ten or fifteen minutes a day of these preliminary exercises/workouts will make a great difference when you later begin your weight training. The routine and regularity of your sessions (remedial or preliminary if you haven't been physically active) will do you a lot of good. Though scorned as old-fashioned, unnecessary or worthless, these kinds of exercise programs can help with the general vigor and health. It may seem as though you are sending yourself to your own basic training or physical education camp, but it's still a good idea, borrowed from the supposedly old-fashioned tradition of physical culture. You will be glad you did this.

A key, though seemingly contradictory, point to remember about this preliminary activity program for building a physical base is that when you begin weight-training as a hard gainer, cease the sports or fitness activities you have been doing in your preliminary program. For the first six or twelve weeks of your weight training, drop the other sports and fitness stuff and concentrate your energies on getting used to your hard gainer training with the weights. You will need your energy to train with and recover from the weights. It will become clearer to you when you do this transition in your training why it's better, if not necessary, to do it this way. Later--perhaps even much later--you might want or be able to re-incorporate some of this sports/fitness training into your schedule.

2. HARD GAINER WEIGHT TRAINING - BODYBUILDING

Now let's get on with the training you want to do, the all-important weight training/bodybuilding for the hard gainer: workouts. The first workout to use is the most basic/beginner's routine for a drug-free trainer or bodybuilder. This workout, or something like it, is often the first routine that many of us have started on in weight-training, bodybuilding or lifting. Though it is considered a basic routine, don't be misled; it can often be very strenuous, depending on how hard the given trainee works on this. And it is true that many strong and well-muscled natural weight-trainers and bodybuilders have made many great gains on such a routine, and either continue to use it or return to it. Exercises and the main muscle area they work are listed. It looks like this:

3. Whole Body Routine, Train Three Times Weekly:

Exercise	Sets	Reps	
Bench Press	1-3	8-12	Chest
Bentover Rowing	1-3	8-12	Back
Behind the Neck Press	1-3	8-12	Shoulders
Curls	1-3	8-12	Biceps
Lying Tricep Extension	1-3	8-12	Triceps
Squats	1-3	8-12	Thighs
Standing Calfraise	1-3	12-20	Calves
Crunch Situps	1-3	8-12	Abs

Begin by doing one set of each exercise and eventually, over a period of workouts, work up to as many as three per exercise, if you can. This is a good workout for hard gainers because it features an all-around approach, as all the major muscle groups are worked, and there is a standard amount of repetitions and a decent range of volume (from one to three sets, a total of from 8 to 24 for the entire workout) to choose from. Sometimes, however, this routine is too tough for hard gainers. If so, you should keep to two or even one set per exercise, but don't train to limit reps (also known as training to failure). Work the set hard for whatever reps you choose to do, then rest a minute or so and do your next set (or exercise). This is a good time to consider two major aspects of weight training: exercise technique, or form, and rest time between sets.

Exercise Technique (Form)

You should always lift any weight safely and under control. You should lift the bar so that it is traveling evenly, smoothly, in a level fashion (as opposed to one side up, one side lagging). There are a number of ways to approach how long a repetition should take, but an almost standard bodybuilding method is to lift the weight in a one-to-two second time span and lower it in the same. If, for example, you are doing a barbell curl, grip the bar in an undergrip (palms facing away from your body as you initially hold the bar) with both hands, with the bar resting across the front of your legs while you stand, with your arms hanging at your sides.

You would smoothly and evenly begin curling the bar upward by curling the bar up and initially away from body, moving only your forearms, keeping your upper arms at your sides with your elbows stationary, then as the bar is raised the arc of the curl will bring the bar up and back toward your body again, so that after one or two seconds the barbell would reach the top of the curl, with the bar being held tightly up near your shoulders. You would then reverse the movement in lowering the bar through the same pathway.

While you will read a lot of variations about exercise form, the point is this: a relatively slow, controlled raising and lowering of the weight is not only safe, but effective. You will be assured of working the targeted muscle (in our example, the biceps), in this way. If you lift too fast or sloppily, and use momentum, or other muscles too much, you will defeat the purpose of trying to work the biceps. This good form is safe and productive, and you can concentrate mentally, focusing on working the biceps. This training style is efficient, effective and safe.

Rest Intervals

After you complete eight repetitions or however many you are doing of a given exercise, and you put the weight down, you have completed a set. How much time before you pick up the weight and do another set, either with the same poundage or a different one? This, too, can vary. But the key for hard gainers is to take a minute or two, or however much time within reason you need to get ready for a quality effort for your next set. You don't want to cool down, and you don't want to let the feeling of blood which has flushed the muscle you are working--the pump--vanish.

You may have heard of, seen or even done workouts where you compress the rest intervals between sets. Instead of the standard one minute (which is a good generalization, though a generalization nonetheless), experienced bodybuilders--often easy gainers, or bodybuilders trying to burn excess bodyfat--will shorten the rest periods to 45 or 30 seconds or less. This method, while productive for them, is not the best one for hard gainers.

Hard gainers, due to their highly sensitive nervous systems, need to rest fully a minute, or two, or three--or perhaps five minutes between sets of heavy squats, bench presses or deadlifts--before they do their next set. This will enable the hard gainer to handle reasonable poundages for him, yet recover enough between sets to give a full effort. Most hard gainer training should be done with regular or longer rest periods between sets, though like most rules, it can be modified carefully as the trainee becomes more proficient. But remember, as a hard gainer, you are trying to build muscle mass and strength, and you do not have much bodyfat to concern yourself with as of this stage of your development.

Poundage Selection & increases—Safety

A word about selecting what weight to use in your exercises. Particularly if you are a beginner, choose conservatively. For example, if you want to do eight repetitions in the squat, and you feel you can handle fifty or one hundred pounds comfortably, then do so. While ideally you should not train alone (you should have a spotter or spotters), safety is paramount. There are racks available with safety stops for bench pressing and squatting, and if you can use these you should be able to train with added peace of mind as far as safety goes.

In addition to basic safety considerations, though, you should not be struggling and straining with poundages. This is an invitation to bad exercise technique, potential injury, and at the very least will guarantee that the targeted muscle area is not being worked correctly. Stop a repetition or two short of what you perceive as your limit, particularly in exercises such as squats and bench presses. And choose poundages that you can handle in good form. Increase your weights over the period of several workouts—don't just pile on the plates, especially if you haven't got that much strength to begin with. Work the exercises diligently and hard--your strength will increase gradually, then you'll be able to handle more weight. And so it goes. Or should, if you do it correctly. Train safely and wisely and you'll reap greater benefits.

Warm ups & Stretching

Along with choosing exercise poundages wisely and using good form in your workouts, you should have a general warm up for a couple of minutes to get your circulation up, your heart rate up, and to loosen up your muscles and joints for the effort to come. Riding a stationary bike, running in place, some light calisthenics will do this. Then, after your body is warmed up, you can do a couple of very light warm up sets with the weights, or you can do one or two of these preceding some of your weight-training sets, particularly on the harder exercises such as squats, bench presses, or deadlifts when you eventually do those. Stretching is best done after our muscles are already warmed up, so although many people stretch first, it is preferable to either do this after your general warm up or perhaps even after your weight training workout. Following these guidelines should help performance and should lessen your chance of injuries.

INJURIES

A quick note here about injuries. You don't want them, but they happen to just about everybody. Whether it's a slight strain or small aches, hard gainers, due to their lighter structures and less hardy constitutions, may suffer more than their share. Always take precautions; injury prevention is far preferable to rehabilitation. As we mentioned, warm up, stretch, work with correct exercise form; pay attention to your exercise habits; take care of your muscles and your body.

If you get small aches or slight injuries, you can carefully try to work lighter, or work around these aches or slight injuries. Avoid exercising that area. You don't want small aches and pains to grow into large chronic pains or injuries. If it becomes more serious, see a physician or therapist. A medical professional who is informed about athletics and bodybuilding can help direct you to beneficial therapies, whether conventional or alternative. Forget the macho thing of working through pain; the bodybuilding journey for you as a hard gainer will be a sustained one. So for longevity and the best results, train safe and smart, with an eye toward protection against injury.

Now we return to our first workout, keeping in mind that some hard gainers can work up to as many as three sets in their initial three times weekly workouts. Some trainees, however, don't recover very well even when the sets are reduced in this workout. If so, then at this point, make the following change:

4. The Twice Weekly Workout

If the workout three times per week is too much, if you feel you aren't progressing, then train only twice per week. Continue to gradually increase your exercise poundages. Instead of, for example, training Monday, Wednesday, and Friday, train only twice each week, for example, Monday and Thursday. Here the initial goal is to continue to make gains but lessen the stress of training. So you may now be training twice per week on one set of each exercise, and using challenging, but not excessive, poundages. Continue to use good form, with a fairly even rep cadence, one or two seconds up and one or two seconds down on each rep. By controlling the weight on the way down each rep, this eccentric/negative portion of the exercise may contribute to muscle growth and strength.

5. Further Reductions

You may also try reducing the reps eventually, to a range of 5 to 8 instead of the initial, standard 8 to 12. You might want to eliminate abdominal work, as most hard gainers don't need it, though you can return to it sometime later. Some have found ab work inhibits gains, and some thin hard gainers trying to eat more have found that ab work sometimes temporarily contracts the stomach area and dampens your immediate desire to eat after training. And we know how important it is for hard gainers to eat.

Layoffs/Training Breaks

Before we go further, now might be a good time to discuss the principle of taking layoffs from training to enhance your results. The nature of bodybuilding or any kind of weight training is that after a period of weeks, usually, the body does not respond as well (or not at all) to training. Your energy will often be lower, and you may not recover from workouts as well. This is the body signaling its response to stress, which can set up the weight-trainer for injuries and illness that further compound the lack of progress. You can fall into a situation then where for long stretches of time you make little or no progress.

To avoid this, you should plan occasional breaks from your training.   Every four, six, eight or twelve weeks--whatever time you determine for yourself--are the usual intervals for training breaks.   Though you may be super-enthusiastic and motivated, sometimes it is simply better to back off from what can be the hard grind of training.   We realize this advice is easier given and understood than followed; if you find you love to train you won't want to take a break, but a break is just what you need for long term progress.

Concentrated/Limited Routine

If the two day a week workout schedule is too much, and, for example, your system still feels drained by Thursday after a Monday workout and you can only squat with twenty or thirty pounds less than your exercise poundage on Monday, then cut back further. You can continue to work out at first twice per week, but try working only the largest of your muscle groups with compound exercises. Use a pressing exercise for your chest and shoulders, a rowing exercise for your back, and squats for your thighs. This, surprisingly, often works when the other workouts don't, though it looks minimal on paper. So you'd have this:

Exercise	Sets	Reps
Bench Press (or Behind the Neck or Overhead Press)	1	5-8
Bentover Row	1	5-8
Squats	1	5-8

Many people will claim to have invented or pioneered this type of workout, but it and its likenesses were around several decades ago. You can try working this twice a week, as we mentioned; the elimination of the other exercises may be enough to provide additional recovery for you to complete this workout more comfortably twice a week than your previous, slightly longer, full-body workout. This type of concentrated routine can work because the major areas of the body for strength and muscle growth are getting stimulated without extraneous work, and you'll have the opportunity for plenty of rest, too.

After a period of time on this routine, you may want to add a set or two, which you may do, but which you should do gradually. You may work up to three sets or so. Some have used more, but save that for later, it's something you might be able to use in the future. Though at first we reduced the amount of training greatly, we are carefully, slowly, increasing it again. But this should be done only if you are adapting to the workload and can handle it. Otherwise, keep your workload more limited. And even if you eventually are able to do three sets per exercise, your workout will still consist of a total of only nine sets, which is approximately what the absolute beginner whole body routine first consisted of. The emphasis here, though, is on the big exercises, so if you continue to work the exercises hard and gradually increase the poundages, you should make gains.

If this workout is not giving you sufficient gains, or is taxing your recovery ability once again, you have two choices. You can cut back on the number of sets again, or you can push the frequency of your training back. Instead of training Monday and Thursday, push the second workout of the week back until Friday, then don't work out again until Tuesday, then Saturday, etc. You have added a rest day for each workout on what began as your twice a week frequency. (Instead of twice in seven days, you will now be working out twice every eight or nine days, on average).

You may keep pushing back your training frequency if you wish to keep experimenting. Working out every fourth or fifth day, or even as infrequently as once every week, sometimes does it as far as promoting gains and ensuring recovery. Some, in extreme cases, may want to reduce the frequency further. Go ahead and experiment with this if you want. Each person's recovery pattern is unique and you need to find these things out for yourself eventually.

6. Extremely Reduced Training

This routine is the result of further moving your training in the direction of less, which will take you to a point where you are doing what amounts to a two-exercise routine. It will consist of:

Bench Press
Squat or Deadlift

Whatever workout frequency you have set for yourself, whether it's once a week (or even less frequent, in some cases), or every fourth, fifth or sixth day, you will be doing the bench press for your upper body and either the squat or deadlift, but not both, for your lower body. The squat and deadlift are actually closer to "whole body" exercises, with their involvement of so many major muscle groups.

While the topic of the benefits of the squat along with or versus the deadlift can be an extensive subject, for our purposes here we should just keep in mind that the squat targets the thighs, buttocks, some lower back and hamstring mainly, whereas the deadlift's effects are felt in the lower back (strongly), the hamstrings, some in the thighs, and even in the upper back, trapezius and shoulders.

The squat and deadlift have a slightly different emphasis, but there is more overlap than you might think. What they both do is vigorously tax the back of the body from the lower back on down, and for some hard gainers, (and even some extremely strong bodybuilders and powerlifters), these exercises represent a partial duplication. They are both, however, fantastic exercises for all-over body power, strength, muscle growth and conditioning. They also, when worked heavily and hard, or for high reps, can be brutally hard. You may even alternate the squats and deadlifts--many trainees do, with excellent results. You can choose the sets and reps yourself; experiment to see what you respond to best and train accordingly. And, despite the minimal nature of these programs, watch your recovery.

7. One Exercise Workout (High Rep Squats--the Legendary Growth Workout)

In the most extreme cases of all, one exercise only, usually the squat, has been used as a total body exercise, and as an entire workout. The benefits of from one to three hard sets of squats, often for reps in the ten to twenty range with a challenging poundage (for that particular trainee), has brought about muscle growth results where everything else has failed. Because the squat places such great demands on the system, the overall body is tremendously stimulated to have a better chance at muscle growth. And while high-rep squatting has come to occupy an almost mythical place in the legends of drug-free bodybuilding, it is not necessarily the cure all for a lack of muscular growth, but for some it has been magic. A little more about that later.

8. High-Rep Deadlifts (The Super Growth Workout)

If you want to try an approach to a super-growth workout, similar to the high-rep squatting, you might venture to try high-rep deadlifts. This can be an extremely difficult workout, but it may result in terrific muscle growth. We have always suggested that the deadlift may be used in place of the squat for the one exercise workout. The deadlift is even more demanding than the squat, which is both its benefit and its potential problem. Some hard gainers have a terrible time handling even respectable poundages in the exercise, and worse times recovering. There are bodybuilders and strength athletes--including some of the strongest powerlifters--who do not train the deadlift directly or often, so take this into account. It is like many other advanced techniques or exercises--some trainees get great results, others mediocre, others none. All you can do is give the program an honest effort and gauge how you'll respond. Be warned, though, a set of ten or twenty reps in the deadlift with a challenging poundage (for you, again, not for someone else) can be extremely draining, even compared to other exercises, and can require even longer recovery periods.

You may find you can only deadlift effectively every ten days or two weeks (or even less often) or so and make progress. Many bodybuilders feel that the effort and energy expenditure weighed against the relatively long recovery time makes the work-result equation unattractive, so they don't utilize the deadlift this way (or, as we said, at all). Others, who respond better or who are able or can adjust their workouts and nutrition to be able to recover, can be rewarded with additional muscle growth, making the effort more than worthwhile. This is an unusual workout, often categorized as one you would use for a period of time such as six to twelve weeks, then return or graduate to a more comprehensive program.

Another one-exercise program, though not very often suggested, consists of the bench press only. The problem with doing benches only is that the upper body is worked for growth, but while the chest, shoulders and arms, along with some of the upper back, get worked thoroughly, you are of course not working the lower body.   So, we're reluctant to recommend this workout, as it can teach the trainee to do relatively easier upper-body work at the expense of leg and back work, which is where most of the body's strength and power potential, as well as potential for muscle growth, is located. But if you are a hard gainer whose build is greatly out of proportion--if your upper body is extremely thin and underdeveloped, yet your lower body--hips and thighs--are relatively more robust, you might do this routine for a while to try to bring your upper body into harmony with your lower body. But remember, the squat and deadlift may make your upper body grow without being worked as directly, whereas obviously the bench press won't do the same for your lower body.   In   times   past,   gyms   were   filled   with disproportionately built bench press/upper body specialists, whose neglect of their back, thighs and hips resulted in a lopsided strength and physique. Be aware of this, then make your choices.

9. One Exercise Rotation Workout

This is a fairly radical workout concept, but one which can produce gains where other methods have failed, also.

You continue to apply the principle of one exercise per workout only, but instead of the squat or deadlift, you would do the bench press one workout, wait a few or several days, depending on how you have previously learned how you personally recover, then do a squat workout, then wait a few or several days, and do a deadlift workout. So it might look like this: Monday, Bench, Thursday, Squat, Monday, Deadlift, Thursday, Bench, etc.

If you find you are doing too much back/hip/leg work via the squat and deadlift, and too little upper body work with the bench press, then simply do the rotation with the Monday workout using the Bench Press, and the Thursday workout one week squatting, the following Thursday the Deadlift. Don't become obsessed with the frequency of the workout so much as the work/recovery principle that is designed to give you hard, concentrated work on a major area of the body (via one exercise at a time), resting, then moving on to another major area.   As opposed to the one set high-rep squat or deadlift workouts, you might try 1-4 sets of as few as 5 or as many as 12 reps for this rotation style workout. It is simply a different stimulus with different reps and sets.

(More About) High Rep Squats & Deadlifts

Done either alone as a workout unto itself or incorporated into a larger workout, the time-honored ten to twenty rep (or more) set of squats can produce great gains, as we have mentioned. So too, in its place, can the deadlift, as we have also mentioned. The growth from these exercises can be great, but you must be prepared to do other workouts sometime later. Despite what some proponents say, doing a workout based on high rep squatting (or deadlifting) is not going to give you infinite gains, continuous strength increases and unlimited muscle growth. Anyone who suggests otherwise is wrong. What these approaches--which are highly intensive workouts--can do, is to promote gains where other things haven't worked, or to boost a lagging rate of progress and growth. Six to twelve weeks--or even less--can be productive, but most people need to move on to another type of workout. You can return to these approaches from time to time, or weave them into an overall workout plan if you wish, but realize that all workouts and nutritional approaches have limitations. The following workout is one such example.

10. Limit Training

One of the most popular styles of workouts in recent years has been the one-set per bodypart, so-called training to failure workout. It goes by various names and has been popularized as "high intensity training" and various other names. This way of working out does have value, and it has some application for hard gainers, though proclaimed as the "only" or "best" way to working out, it falls short. This is not the place to fully debate the merits of the approach, but the short story is that the great effort required is sometimes too much for hard gainers (as well as everyone else).

When you train to the last rep you can possibly do on a given set (your limit rep or the "failure" in training to failure), it exacts a tremendous toll on the nervous system. Recovery and growth--no matter what you do in terms of restricting the training amount or how long you rest between workouts--may be severely compromised. Hard gainers tend to have poor recovery ability to begin with, and nervous systems that don't react well to this kind of effort/neural "overload" in the first place.

It is, despite the prevailing nearly universal view in bodybuilding today, possible to overwork via working too hard on a given set. Try this style of workout for a while--carefully. You may gain on it for a couple of weeks, or not at all, or you may be one of the rare ones for whom this style is totally suited. To modify, go to near-limit reps; this is the secret of making brief, intensive workouts work (despite what its loudest proponents claim): not burning your nervous system reserves out on one set, one rep or one workout, but working hard yet still conserving such energy.

11. Change: "Graduating" to Other Routines

One of the things most hard gainers need to do and often fail to do, is to change their workouts from these brief, limited routines when they have become sufficiently accustomed to the workload, and/or have stopped gaining, to other routines. Traditional hard gainer advice often insists that hard gainers forever stay on limited routines, but the originators of such routines in the long ago, nearly forgotten days of bodybuilding, often did not, nor did they recommend that. Even the routines for which spectacular claims are made, such as high-rep squatting or the limited whole body routine, are not appropriate for the best gains for hard gainers forever.

The body often responds to one style of workouts, whether it is heavy weights or moderate weights with volume, higher or lower reps, by growing, but after a time (which can be a highly individualized period of time), the trainee often stops growing muscle, and the bodybuilder may become overtrained. This can happen more often and more easily with hard gainers than with regular trainers, as the hard gainer's system tends to react much more sensitively to the stress of whatever workout they are on. Yet the majority of advice given for hard gainers is by far to keep plugging away on the same limited routine, even for years. It's as if at some point muscle growth and/or strength is going to kick in and the hard gainer will begin to make gains, whether a little, or a lot. The truth is that staying with the same program often brings futility, or if it has been successful, limits further gains.

Vary Your Training (& The Value of Conditioning)

All bodybuilders and athletes usually need to do this more, but for hard gainers, it can be essential. The hard gainer needs to change his training. He can return to heavy weights (for him) and a more limited program in the future, but he may need to see if he can now do a two or three day a week whole body routine, even if he originally was unable to do so. By having concentrated on a limited routine, he should have conditioned his body to be able to train better, so the whole body routine, while he might need to adjust to it, may be much more do-able and even result producing for him.

The value of conditioning and overall fitness levels as a contribution to overall muscle growth is often neglected by natural bodybuilders, almost always by hard gainers. This is a critical and overlooked move for almost all hard gainers, so much so that it can almost be considered a secret, since so few do it and understand it. It is also important to adjust the whole body routine. Moderate, not heavy, poundages should be used, for 8-12 reps per set. There will be a slight training volume increase, coupled with perhaps a slightly lighter or less intensive workload. This will enable the hard gainer to adjust and probably gain, where before he could not.

12. Volume: Carefully Increased Sets & Reps

The reason you'll be able to do slightly more volume (sets and reps) than when you began is that your body has become somewhat conditioned to working out. And although recovery ability--including the ability to handle a longer routine, doesn't often dramatically change for an individual (as much as, for example, strength and muscle size may), simply working out for a number of months or years does improve this somewhat.

We emphasize again that general fitness and conditioning is important for all bodybuilders (and is usually neglected), but it is vital to the health and potential progress of hard gainers.   So, when adding volume, add it gradually, carefully, and don't go overboard. Don't start training like an easy gainer who can add lots of sets, reps and exercises and still make gains and recover. But do attempt to increase your work capacity along with your ability to train harder.

Why add reps and sets? You will give a decidedly different stimulus to the muscles. A different rep scheme, usually higher, with lighter or moderate poundages, often works better once some muscle and strength is gained, especially in the case of hard gainers. Your body has become somewhat accustomed to working out and it does not react with the near-shock reaction of your early days of training (remember your first attempts at working out?). Slightly higher reps and a few more additional sets work the muscles--their fibers and other constituent parts--differently than low reps or heavier poundages. Your key as a hard gainer is to put yourself under a measured type of stress during your workout, not to throw everything in at once.

You may find if you have been stagnant on one of the limited routines, that returning to a full body routine two or three times a week with, for example, 2 sets of 12 reps and relatively moderate poundages (less weight than you were using on your more limited routine), gives you some additional gains.

Further Modifications: Exercise Changes (Towards Complete Development)

In a very controlled way, a hard gainer may now add or occasionally substitute some isolation exercises. Most hard gainer advisors suggest trainees leave these alone. But isolation exercises, (sometimes called "shaping exercises") can be used judiciously, and they can be necessary as well, since full shape and development can be difficult or even impossible if a bodybuilder only relies on basic exercises all the time. And while "isolation" is an imprecise, relative term, there are some excellent exercises in that category that can benefit a typical hard gainer.

If a hard gainer is doing a basic workout, six to eight exercises, one to three sets each, two days per week, and is recovering sufficiently, perhaps he can add a third workout which includes more isolation work. During this workout, he could utilize a "mass-shape" strategy, which would include what are nearly hybrid exercises (contributing both, nearly equally to overall mass and shape), such as incline bench presses instead of the regular flat bench press, etc. or more fully isolation-shaping moves such as flyes, lateral raises, etc. Or, you can occasionally substitute these exercises for your main, basic ones from time to time.

13. Mass-Shape Routine/Exercises

Incline Bench Press	Chest
Upright Rows	Shoulders
Lat Pulldowns	Back
Dumbbell Curls	Biceps
Seated Tricep Extensions	Triceps
Front Squats	Thighs
Donkey Calfraise	Calves
Leg Raise	Abs

These exercises--and the list is not exhaustive--give a combination of mass and shape that is slightly different than the basic exercises you've used. These exercises tend to work the large muscle groups with a different emphasis than the basic exercises. Further shaping/development can be achieved through the use of the following routine. Remember, as in the previous routine, to either incorporate these exercises as occasional substitutes for your basic ones, or to do perhaps one of every three workouts or so using these. The mass-shape exercises in the previous list can be used more often than these exercises, which are less mass and more isolation oriented. These isolation/shaping moves are very much supplementary, occasional and adjunctive, more so than even the mass/shape routine.

Isolation-Shaping Routine/Exercises
(very occasional/substitutional)

Flyes	Chest
Lateral Raises	Shoulders
Chin-ups	Back
Preacher Curls	Biceps
Tricep Pressdowns	Triceps
Hack Squats	Thighs
Angled Calfraise	Calves
One-quarter situp	Abs

Don't be concerned if you don't have the equipment to do the exact exercises. You can simply search or choose to find exercises that work the same general muscle area (chest, for example) but that work a different area or emphasis. These types of workouts or the inclusion of these exercises can comprise a certain percentage of more accomplished bodybuilders' workouts, but hard gainers, while eventually including them, should always carefully monitor the effect.

If you begin to overtrain or progress halts, revert to your more basic routines, those which by now should have been successful for you. By now, you should have trained enough on standard hard gainer (three times a week) workouts or the more limited workouts, and you should be well versed in what works for you. In this way when you experiment, you'll always have something to fall back on that has worked for you in the past.

14. Progressive Change (Continuous Change; Progression)

Even though you are a hard gainer, there are some things you can mimic which are beneficial for easier gaining bodybuilders. One of these is "progression". As applied to most bodybuilding, progression usually is used to refer only to "progressive resistance,"i.e., adding weight to the bar, so the bodybuilder who begins by doing repetitions with, say, 30 pounds in the curl works his way up to 50 or 65 or however many pounds. This is the most basic way of progressing and is valuable, though often it becomes a one-dimensional, limited application.

Hard gainers are often told that increasing their exercise poundages is the only way they can gain muscle size. But this is not the case. For one thing, beyond the beginner's stage, adding weight to the bar on a linear basis doesn't continue indefinitely--or for very long, without plateau or periods of stagnation. Strength fluctuates; more so for the hard gainer. One day you may be able to lift 30 pounds for, say, eight reps in the curl, then in a couple of weeks 35 and 40 pounds for 8 reps, for example, then the week after that your strength may regress to 35 pounds or even back to 30 pounds again for 8 reps and remain stagnant (or fall off further) for several weeks. This fluctuation, this difficulty, despite what many experts claim, is nearly universal and becomes more difficult as you progress.

So do this: begin with the standard workout, make whatever reductions or slight increases you need to. Gradually add (or add back) a slight amount of volume, reps or sets (not both at once); if you have to cut back for a while after this, do so, then continue making changes and additions. You can add isolation workouts or exercises, and so on.

Volume, variety, different exercises, different set and rep schemes--all these tactics are employed by average and easy gaining drug-free bodybuilders to build muscle size and strength, and so they should be employed by you, in a more controlled way, as a hard gainer. To do otherwise is to possibly limit your results.

Other Advanced Training Techniques (Greater Workout Changes)

There are many other training techniques, usually referred to as intensity techniques, which increase the effort, if not the result of workouts. These are such things as supersets, down-the-rack, forced reps, training to failure (limit reps, discussed earlier), negative reps (eccentric training), partial reps, lock-outs, supports, and so on. While these techniques can be useful for many natural bodybuilders, they are often overused. The misguided belief that you cannot train too hard or too heavy and therefore overtrain, but that you can overtrain only on how much training you can do, does not represent the reality of how the human body works. So, not only are easy gaining bodybuilders using these techniques too often, but hard gainers need to be very cautious about their use.

There is just no sense in doing something in training that causes you to overtrain or injure yourself or to abruptly cause your progress to cease. Try these types of techniques experimentally, and extremely infrequently. If you can use them productively, fine. If not, the other, more standard methods of straight sets, gradual changes in exercises, sets, reps and workouts, along with other progressive changes, should give you the type of progress you seek without burning you out, injuring you, or wrecking your health.

III. RECOVERY

1. How to Improve Your Gains

Though technically we have concentrated on the two major areas of bodybuilding, nutrition and training, there is a third major area of importance: recovery. This is a much-neglected area, and is usually given cursory attention or a typically one-dimensional approach. Easy gainers tend to ignore recovery, by and large, in factoring in their bodybuilding. More average-potential drug-free bodybuilders usually consider recovery only when they have massively overtrained or have injured themselves, or progress has stopped on a long-term basis. Hard gainers are told, perhaps, to work out on a much more limited basis and "watch their recovery"--decent advice as far as it goes, but this can be expanded. Monitoring your results, energy and recovery is a good start, but including recovery in your initial planning of your bodybuilding in the first place and then paying attention all the way along might eventually pay bigger dividends.

Recovery Strategy

What you can do is include some practical actions to adjust your recovery as part of the overall equation of your bodybuilding. The first thing usually recommended, of course, is to reduce the frequency or severity of your workouts if you are not recovering or gaining. That is to say, what you should not do is too much or work out with too much weight or intensity, and so on, for you to recover. But you should also attempt, as we have shown, to gradually get into better shape so that despite your need to initially do perhaps only very brief workouts, eventually to build up your conditioning so you can at least do a little more. This is controversial among experts; few feel that hard gainers can increase recovery ability, but better eating (more calories as opposed to fewer when you started), and building up your muscular system (endurance) and getting your nervous system used to the exertion of bodybuilding/weight-training can improve your ability to handle more work.

Your general physical conditioning is a factor in not just your body's ability to handle the workouts, but to recover from them, and therefore is important for your bodybuilding training and results. It's likely true that recovery ability in this way is highly genetically factored, and the range of improvement will be less than, say, your potential to increase strength or gain muscle size, even if you're a hard gainer, but even slight improvement is worthwhile.

Other Physical Activity

At least in the beginning stages of your hard gainer program, you should seriously consider confining your sports/fitness/physical activity to your weight-training workouts only. If your recovery ability is poor--and it almost certainly is--you need to conserve your energy for your weight workouts and for recovering from them. If you expend further energy playing sports one or two days per week in addition to your bodybuilding workouts, you may lose what little muscle and strength you have, and at best you may prevent any gains.

Particularly deadly in this regard are aerobics: running, jogging, treadmill, playing basketball--any form of aerobics, which while potentially beneficial for health and athletics, at this stage of your training, they will almost certainly be detrimental to your bodybuilding gains. You need to build up your energy reserves and you need not to burn up precious calories with these types of activities. We realize that this path is sometimes difficult to follow, but at least attempt to eliminate or severely restrict this type of outside activity for the first six to twelve weeks of your program.

Give your body a chance to grow into a gaining phase--gain weight, muscle size and strength--before you decide to eventually include or return to any outside activity. You may eventually include such activity in a controlled way from time to time along with your workouts. But always monitor your bodybuilding progress and be prepared to adjust (downward) any outside physical activity if you have to. For hard gainers, even if you train for years, you should always carefully monitor extra/extraneous activity. That's what it is if your main interest is in bodybuilding.

2. Synergy of Recovery

You can better adjust your eating to match the severity and duration of your workouts. If you're doing a high-rep squatting routine within a three-times weekly full body workout, you should consider pushing your calories over what you've been eating on a standard routine. But don't gorge yourself. And yes, while we've advocated pushing back the workout frequency (sometimes radically so), to get more rest days--sometimes many more--this strategy, too, has its limits.

Sleep and Rest

Sleep is a huge, overlooked recovery factor, given a society in which the minimum amount of sleep possible seems prevalent. Regular sleep each night—eight hours or however much you need--can be crucial to your bodybuilding. Elite athletes (and old-time bodybuilders and weight-lifters) know that an added half-hour of sleep or extra hour, or a short nap (or two!), can do a great deal to restore/enhance energy. Often, only the absence of sleep is noticed by athletes and bodybuilders, once they have abused and neglected this for a long time, the cumulative insult shows itself in poor bodybuilding results. The workout or trainer or diet or something else is often blamed.

Rest and relaxation are often neglected, and can be more subtle even than sleep. Again, their absence, rather than their inclusion as a positive principle, are more noted. If you work at a stressful job which you hate, for forty to sixty hours a week, are constantly tired, don't sleep well or eat well or can't relax, have little time or energy for enjoyable activities, have poor relationships, and an unhappy life, what you are doing in your bodybuilding workouts as a hard gainer is going to be far more difficult to succeed with than if you have the opportunity to have a better balanced, happier life where work does not totally deplete you, where you are happy and fulfilled outside your work in your personal life, where you can eat and rest well, where you have friends and people you care about and who care about you, and you generally look forward to each day rather than wishing it would all go away. But all this is considered to be beyond the province of bodybuilding.

Keep trying to effect an improved composite of your bodybuilding: training, nutrition, recovery, attitude, etc. None of these things alone will transform you from a hard gainer into a superman, but taken together, they can contribute mightily to enhancing your results. There is a synergy here: small bits of improved recovery, which don't seem like much, can add up to a great deal.

3. How to Advance

As a hard gainer, just as anyone else, your rate of progress and eventual results will be individualized, which is simply to say that your progress and results will most likely be different from the next person's, even if that person is a fellow hard gainer. That said, however, once you have applied much of the information we've given here, you should have made progress--not without difficulties and setbacks, we understand, but progress nevertheless. Where as a beginning hard gainer, perhaps you had to reduce your workout load and increase your eating, which likely triggered your gains. You may have run into setbacks when you tried to train too much for your system's recovery at that time, but then over a period of a several months or even a couple of years, surprised yourself with the muscle and strength you have gained. Congratulations--the effort and results are yours!

You may have even developed the ability to handle more and harder work and you feel you want to progress beyond the many routines and the way we've outlined your training here. While many who teach about hard gainer bodybuilding would discourage this, progressing, and sometimes even in the workload, can be very beneficial. Just remember to be honest in monitoring your results, energy and commitment, so that if you have to backtrack, do so. Don't worry about it. It's all about making the best training, nutrition and results for you, and fitting it all into your life, not someone else's.

4. ADVANCED HARD GAINER WORKOUTS

If you have gone through some or all or even a few of the workout schedules we've detailed, and you've handled them and want to try to do a little more, this is where you might want to aim: instead of the less frequent training, which has been roughly from once per week (or even less often) to three times per week, you can try a split routine, where you work out four days per week. You would do this (as an example):

Exercise	Sets	Reps
Monday, Thursday (Chest, Shoulders, Arms)		
Bench Press	1-3	8-12
Seated Behind the Neck Press	1-3	8-12
Curls	1-2	8-12
Lying Tricep Extensions	1-2	8-12
(Abs optional)		
Tuesday, Friday (Legs & Back)		
Squats	1-3	8-12
Calfraise	1-3	8-12
Deadlifts (Tuesday only)	1-3	8-12
Rows (Friday only)	1-3	8-12
(Abs optional)		

Average or easy gainers would look at this schedule and say, "so what, big deal, it isn't very much work," (if they would even be that charitable), but for many true hard gainers, this four days per week two-way split is a major foray into challenging territory. Keep the sets down at first, gradually get into this, then if you feel you are handling the workload and progressing, add a set or two slowly. Remember, many hard-gainer trainers/coaches tell you to stay on only the most limited routines. Here, if you can effectively do these routines --which are used by many better gaining bodybuilders—and recover, your gains might be greater. Some hard gainers continue to gain on very limited programs, and this is what their systems tolerate best or only, for as long as they may train, which may be many years. That's fine. You may get great results that way. Again, it is an individual matter.

But if you are able to and decide to do this four day workout--which is edging into the workout territory of average gaining natural bodybuilders--you may eventually be able to exploit its great versatility. You may go to lower reps eventually, using 5 to 8 reps per set instead of the standard, initial 8 to 12. You may be able to occasionally substitute some other exercises, for example, on one leg workout you may do parallel squats, then perhaps you'll want to try front squats or high-bar Olympic squats on the other. The key is to stay with exercises that work enough muscle to give you mass gains, even if they have some different effect in shape, proportion and the look of your overall physique.

Plugging in the many variables you might be able to use can give you a lot of options in your workouts, more than you have in the more restricted, necessarily limited formats you might have been using. Or, you can use this four-day workout for a month or six weeks, then return to a three or two times workout for a while--whatever suits you, whatever helps you progress. Vary the amount of workout stress throughout a year; work out harder for a while, then back off, then go harder again, etc. The human body is complex and dynamic, it is not static, not simple, not a machine, where continual hard training can be forced for progress.

On this four day workout, you might try to add a little bit of volume, either through reps and/or sets (for example, three or even four sets of ten, though that's a lot of volume for most). If you find it's too much, simply cut back to where your system can handle it. And again, if you feel you make better gains on briefer work, go with that. Your hard gainer bodybuilding should not be an exercise in slavishly sticking to someone's imposed workout philosophy that is unsuitable for you.   Eventually, through your own experience, you should become the best judge of what is best for you.

5. Strength Training For Hard Gainers

One of the problems with hard gainers is that they initially most often (always?) don't have much strength, and though some would say this equals bodybuilding failure and others might say the lack of strength is irrelevant, these views miss the point. (And yes, there is not a strict, exact correspondence between strength and muscle, despite what the vast amount of oversimplified information you might hear suggests.)   But often this basic lack of strength interferes with the simple performance with even modest poundages for hard gainers. Whether they are interested in strength or not, and putting aside the bodybuilding world's often confused views on the relationships of strength to muscle size and developing it, simply put, hard gainers need to develop some basic strength.

Where the traditional hard gainer programs often run into trouble are when they try to make a hard gainer work out in a modified power program, which would be suitable for an already stronger bodybuilder, and the hard gainer, though he tries mightily, fails on the program or gets injured. Forced reps, training to failure, low reps or dropping a skinny, untrained hard gainer into a powerlifting or even a modified power training or even power bodybuilding workout right at the outset usually doesn't work. If, however, after months or a year or two of successful training, where the hard gainer has learned how to handle the stress of using the weights, and has gained some bodyweight, muscle and at least some level of additional strength, then strength training can work.

6. Hard Gainer Strength Workout

Hard Gainer Strength Workout (Twice Per Week)		
Monday		
Bench Press		
a set of 5 reps, a set of 3 reps, a set of 2 reps		
Squat		
a set of 5 reps, a set of 3 reps, a set of 2 reps		
Deadlift		
a set of 5 reps, a set of 3 reps, a set of 2 reps		
Thursday		
	Sets	Reps
Bench Press	2-3	6-4
Seated Behind the Neck Press	1-2	6-8
Rows	2-3	6-4
Curls	1-2	6-8
Lying Tricep Extensions	1-2	6-8
Squats	2-3	6-4
Calfraise	1-2	8-12

These are very tough workouts. Warm up thoroughly, make sure you do some lighter weight sets before you proceed to your heavier weights. Don't go to limit reps/failure. Make your final rep one in which you could probably do one or two more. Use spotters and/or safety equipment (i.e., safety racks, etc.).

The Thursday workout, with from 10 to 17 total sets, can be taxing to your stamina and conditioning. Reduce the armwork, calfwork, and rowing if you have to. Or, as an alternative, just do the benches, rows and squats on Thursday (6-9 sets total workout) and move the arm and calfwork to a brief Friday or Saturday workout (3-6 total work sets). Be adaptable, and do what you can to preserve this amount of work. If you can't do it all, as we said, then cut back.

This workout will develop strength, some muscle--yes, low reps can develop muscle, even with (or especially with) hard gainers. And even in the unlikely event that handling some heavier poundages for lower reps doesn't give you great mass gains (at first), the ability to handle more weight will be transferable when you switch back to your more customary routines with 8-12 reps or whatever you were using. Everybody is different enough so that they may respond differently. Some hardgainers, however, once they find they are able to handle low reps and develop some strength, make their greatest gains and utilize these types of workouts almost exclusively. Others flourish on higher reps, fewer sets.

7. Big Three Times Three

This workout is similar to the concentrated/limited routine in early part of the hard gainer report, where you would use the Bench Press, Squat, and Deadlift (and Bentover Rowing)--only three exercises per workout, but in this case we will do this workout three times per week, and for some additional sets. It will look like this:

Big Three Times Three		
Monday, Wednesday, Friday		
	Sets	Reps
Bench Press	3-5	5
Squats	3-5	5
Deadlifts (Monday only)	3-5	5
Rows (Wednesday & Friday)	3-5	5

Easy gainers or even average gaining bodybuilders who can handle a large workload might not appreciate this workout, but it can be extremely demanding, not just for hard gainers, but for many other bodybuilders as well. Working the "Big Three," the powerlifts, in a power-bodybuilding format like this, is challenging and should produce great results. If the three workouts are too many, cut back to two. Similarly, if the sets are too much, do the same.

But if you have advanced as a hard gainer, doing this workout which concentrates on where the muscle and power is located most in the body, and eliminating (temporarily) armwork, calfwork, and any overlapping work (shoulders get worked indirectly but hard in this workout), you may grow greatly--even in those areas not directly worked. This workout ultimately can be modified in terms of sets and reps, even for hard gainers, by later concentrating on slightly higher reps and the big exercises, muscle mass increases may be pronounced. A long overlooked workout, regarded as too simple, the big three times three can do wonders for hard gainers.

Revisiting Other Workouts, Other Techniques

When discussing the exercise techniques and workouts for hard gainers as we have, we discouraged the use of training to failure (limit reps), along with intensity techniques, such as supersets, negatives, etc. The matter of conditioning the hard gainer and building up to the effort and necessary systemic recovery that is required to effectively use such things is what our goal was. Once the hard gainer has successfully demonstrated to himself that he can do certain workouts and approaches, he can keep trying more difficult, advanced, and what we hope will be result-producing workouts and techniques.

Limit Training Revisited

So many people believe and practice this form of training, and we acknowledge that for some it is productive. Most hard gainers have a difficult time with it, even when they have progressed to more volume, or through some strength training, and so on. No worthwhile method, however, should be dismissed out of hand. If the hard gainer who has gained weight, strength, muscle mass and is used to applying and recovering from greater intensity wants to try training to failure/limit reps, he should do so. But be forewarned, again, that most hard gainers do not usually do very well on this. We strongly suggest a modification.

Limited/Brief Training

While this seems the same as all-out training to failure, it isn't. If a hard gainer chooses to do a one-set or two-set per bodypart routine, using basic exercises such as those found in our beginner's or usual hard gainer routine, i.e., benches, squats, etc., we strongly suggest again he might get dramatically better results than by training to failure by stopping one or two reps short of that. The combination of the higher reps along with, for the hard gainer, a relatively heavy exercise poundage, is the real benefit of this type of workout, not the act of going to the end of your energy reserves in a set. That is what is most misunderstood.

For example, one or two sets of 10 to 12 reps on the bench press might yield results now whereas when the hard gainer first began, to do 10 or 12 reps might have necessitated very modest or even minuscule poundages. But now, for the hard gainer, the limited, brief approach will preserve recovery energy, and not going to failure will preserve far more central nervous system recovery ability (workout won't be as taxing), but the high reps with a moderate, or for the hard gainer, still heavy poundage (within a rep or two of his limits), will provide a combined intensity without diminishing too much energy--the energy, effort, result equation almost certainly will be far more favorable than training to failure.

Far fewer injuries, far less overtraining, far better recovery will ensue from this modified brief training. For some hard gainers, this kind of approach can become their main workout method, so successful can it become.

Intensity Techniques

For the hard gainer who can handle some strength work and four day workouts (some volume, etc.), he can carefully include, every so often, such things as negatives or supersets or whatever advanced technique that is productive. Still use these sparingly. You can overtrain on one hard work set, though virtually everybody in bodybuilding disagrees with this statement. A negative, partner assisted bench press with a maximum-plus poundage, for example, for one set of a few reps can completely wipe out someone whose system is not used to nor capable of handling it. We're not trying to discourage you or keep you away from productive techniques, just be prudent in your use of them. And should you experience overtraining or injuries, simply rest, get well, and go back to the types of workouts that have worked for you.

8. Getting Back to Basic Training--Reconditioning The Hard Gainer

Another area to re-visit is additional exercise. One of the first things many ambitious hard gainers have to do is cut back other physical activity. Those who have been athletic prior to weight-training often have to be encouraged to cut back or eliminate swimming or running or tennis or whatever it is they have been used to doing. While admittedly great activities, these things burn up a lot of precious hard gainer energy, as well as plenty of hard gainer calories, and potential pounds of bodyweight and muscle.

There is, however, great value in these sports and activities. They help condition the body for effort, they have beneficial cardiovascular effects, and though this is largely irrelevant for hard gainers, they can be helpful (though they are overrated in this way) for fat loss. There is another avenue, though, where these activities help. Conditioning, as we said, is major avenue of importance.

The hard gainer who has done these activities or played these sports and then begins weight training, though not many trainers/coaches/teachers seem to understand this, has a distinct advantage over his non-athletic hard gainer counterpart. Good effects to the metabolism, nervous system, internal organs, and yes, if done right, health-promoting effects may come out of these activities. The fitness craze of simply using exercise as a weight-loss tool, and an overrated one at that, completely misses the value of such activities.

So, if other activities are beneficial, but the hard gainer has limited energy, how do we incorporate them? At first, as we said, after a conditioning period, drop all other activity to enter the initial stages of hard gainer training. Then, after several weeks, months or a couple of years even, if you want to wait that long, you may carefully add them back in. If you are working out three days a week on hard gainer weight training, and have increased your muscle mass, bodyweight and strength, you might want to try on one of your off-days (from the weights) an activity of your choice: jogging, treadmill, swimming--again, your choice.

You can do these things for as little as five, ten or fifteen minutes and they will be beneficial. Do not emulate someone with unlimited energy who will do the treadmill or bike for an hour on the day they're not weight-training. It's likely this will immediately throw you into overtraining, you'll lose muscle mass, weight and strength if you keep it up. But you can do a little bit.

Conditioning Extras: Micro-Workouts

- Five minutes of interval training (sprint/walk/sprint)

- Ten or fifteen minutes on the stationary bike or treadmill

- A brisk twenty or thirty minute walk

- Ten or fifteen minutes of playing basketball, soccer

- Stretching, yoga (this you can do without compromising recovery energy)

- Run a mile (a brisk pace; don't jog)

These are just some examples. The list could be endless; find something you enjoy. If you take periodic layoffs from the weights, you can do more of these sports/activities when you're not doing your hard gainer training. You might lose a slight amount of weight, muscle or strength, but when you return, you'll probably make faster, better progress.

Some hard gainers who have either voluntarily (though not usually) or been forced by circumstances (more likely) to take an entire summer away from the weights, kept up and improved their conditioning doing calisthenics or running or working a physical job and have been surprised when they returned to the weights, even if they have lost some of their gains, how quickly they retrieve them and surpass them. And this other, non-weight-training exercise you do is always ultimately beneficial. (This used to be a staple of weight-training and hard gaining instructions, as people lifted weights with the purpose of eventually using the newfound muscle, strength and vitality in other sports and activities).

These types of exercises and activities are also beneficial if you feel your general conditioning has slipped despite having kept up with your weight-training workouts. This could be considered a kind of remedial conditioning. The addition, however slight, of an activity/exercise other than the weight-training will soon improve and return your conditioning. The different type of exercise from weight-training will ultimately be complementary to your hard gainer training. Everything worthwhile contributes to your overall physical improvement.

Where You Go From Here

If you learn and apply the information we have offered, you can begin to make substantial muscle and strength gains as a hard gainer. Even if you have not had satisfactory results before, now you should be able to find one or several techniques or practical ideas which can help you. Remember, you can improve your eating right from the start, and begin to give your body the nutrients and calories it needs for you to train and recover successfully from training.

If you employ additionally a strategy of activating, watching and even enhancing your recovery, along with your nutritional and training approaches, you may surprise yourself with the type of bodybuilding progress which you didn't think was available to you. Keep training hard and consistently, and keep learning. The elusive goal of your great physique as a hard gainer will come nearer and nearer to you through all your proud efforts.

Ten Growth Principles for Hard Gainers

1. More food. Hard gainers almost universally need to eat more.

2. The right workout (a productive one). Hard gainers need to get on a good general workout, then constantly monitor this to match their training to their present level of both ability & needs.

3. Recovery. This also needs to be matched to meet the training stress and consciously monitored, adjusted, and even worked at (developed).

4. Progressive workouts. There is a need for changing the workouts (in volume, intensity, etc.) and principles to further challenge yourself once the basic or limited routines are successfully undertaken or completed.

5. Take care of your health. This is the foundation for any successful bodybuilding you want to do. Whatever your health profile, monitor it & take care of problems; enhance & improve your health if you can.

6. Build a physical base. This is a much-neglected phase of hard gainer training. Your results will be better both initially

and long term if you have something to work with in this regard (i.e., overall fitness, a background of physical activity, exercise and/or sports). Do not neglect overall conditioning at any time.

7. Train hard, train consistently. For those who do so, this becomes second nature, but some have difficulty sticking to a workout program. It is, however, essential for success that you do.

8. Train across the spectrum. What this simply means is that you need to eventually try other training principles than those you began with, so you can see what ultimately is going to work for you & what isn't.

9. Individualize your nutrition. Just as you need to adjust your training, you are not going to flourish on someone else's eating plan. You need to find the types of foods, balance of nutrients and quantities which are going to be compatible with your health, and will bring you the best bodybuilding results.

10. Train for overall muscle and shape, not just strength. Use poundages you can handle and pay attention the effects on your physique from the various exercises and workouts you'll do. Don't struggle with too-heavy weights and neglect balance, shape and proportion in your physique. This is bodybuilding, not just strength training.

Additional Hard Gainer Tips

1. If you're not gaining, look to your diet. Make sure to eat enough good food; always keep this in mind.

2. If you're still not gaining, check your workout. Are you doing too much? When in doubt, reduce your workout slightly. You can always add back later.

3. Try to build some basic strength. This is what most hard gainers lack, at least initially, yet it can eventually contribute to your mass gains.

4. Learn to focus. All successful bodybuilders know that concentrating on the exercises produces better results. Practice this.

5. Build up your conditioning. Whether it's through using a slightly greater amount of weight in your exercises, or slightly increased reps or volume, or very carefully added and controlled non-weight-lifting physical conditioning, this will help you handle the workload in your workouts.

6. Learn everything you can about training and how your body responds to it. It's your body. Take responsibility for it.

7. If you have progressed, you may add advanced techniques (supersets, forced reps, etc.), but carefully, and you'll be able to benefit.

8. Continue to change your training, yet, though it seems contradictory, if something always works for you, you can keep using it; if something never does, don't keep using it.

9. Alter your eating. After you've gained, change your nutrition to more or less eating depending on your new needs. Always monitor this.

10. Attitude--stay active, positive and patient. Stay persistent, keep training, overcome obstacles, persevere through difficulties, and eventually you'll come through it to make substantial hard gainer progress.

Hard Gainer Frequently Asked Questions

1. Can hard gainers do workouts longer than the ones described here?

A Yes, in some instances, there are hard gainers who develop greater increases in recovery ability than others. Most will still need to cut back to shorter workouts after a while, though.

2. How much muscle can I eventually gain? How strong will I be?

A. No one can predict this. The more extremely thin and un-athletic you are, your potential will be less; if you are thin but not extremely so, you should have better genetics for ultimate growth. Wise training and effort ultimately will influence results.

3. I like to ride my bike and play basketball. Can I still gain size?

A.Yes, but you are very likely going to have to restrict these activities in terms of both duration and frequency. If you notice your strength and size gains halting or reversing, cut back or out on the bike and basketball.

4. My Dad and brother are both thin. Can I overcome these genetics?

A. It's hard to say in advance. People in the same family usually have similar genetics, but there can be enough differences to make the potentials of each for bodybuilding or weight-lifting different. Again, see question #2.

5. I'm an easy gainer, can I use the workouts you recommend for hard gainers?

A. Yes. This is a secret of many easy and average gainers. From time to time, they will cut back to briefer or special workouts such as you find in this book, and this will boost gains as well as often cure overtraining.

6. I try to eat to gain size, but I get flabby yet still am thin.

A. The bane of hard gainers, "skinny fat". You need to work out on the briefer, harder workouts, and adjust your diet to an amount that gains lean muscle mass. You may not even necessarily be a true hard gainer, you may be a more mesomorphic (easy gainer) who hasn't worked out or eaten properly for your body type.

7. I've been working out for several months, but my gains have stopped. What should I do?

A. Assuming you are a true hard gainer (see question #6), you need to assess whether you need a layoff, whether you need to cut back on your workout, or eat more, or some combination of these. These variables are usually the keys to success.

8. Aren't 90% of the drug-free bodybuilders really hard gainers? Isn't the term a cop out?
A. Absolutely not! Hard gainers, as we use the term, are perhaps 10-15% of the drug-free bodybuilders. The term is meaningless as it is now used by many, who claim that "90% of drug-free bodybuilders are hard gainers or average gainers."   This tells you nothing. So the term is a very useful identification and teaching tool, far from a cop out.

9. Will this work for women? Is there anything different I should do?
A. The hard gainer routines and nutrition will work equally well for women. The language in the report is not meant to be gender bound. Thin women who follow these workouts and nutrition often have far better results than men. Some different shaping—hips and weaker upper body should be factored in though in designing a woman's workout.

10. I've come up with my own workout from the principles you advocate. Is this okay?
A. It's great. I assume it works. Always, individualized, customized workouts—those that work best for you, especially hard gainers—become the best workouts.

A Simple Blender Drink:

(The staple of hard gainer "extra" nutrition or supplementation, you can make your own weight-gain/muscle-gain drink inexpensively).

Mix/blend:
- ✓ whole milk
- ✓ banana
- ✓ honey (½ teaspoon, for flavor)

  you can add:
- ✓ 2 lightly boiled eggs (instead of raw eggs)
- ✓ protein powder (or powdered milk)
- ✓ half n half (boosts calories)

Good luck to all hard gainers in your training!

ABOUT GREG SUSHINSKY

Greg Sushinsky is a longtime natural bodybuilder and writer whose work has appeared in leading bodybuilding magazines for years. He has competed as a bodybuilder as well as a powerlifter, continues to train hard while also writing and instructing on bodybuilding. He is the author and publisher of The Natural Bodybuilding Training Manual, as well as The Hard Gainer Report. As a professional writer, his other work has been published extensively in mainstream sports magazines, as well as numerous fitness and health publications. He lives with his wife in the Cleveland, Ohio area.

Visit Greg's website, **Premier Bodybuilding**
at www.gregsushinsky.com